I0441496

Software
For
diabetics

ROBERT STETSON

ISBN: 978-1481993395

TABLE OF CONTENTS

PREFACE

The software in this book can be easily downloaded and installed from my website. The URL (Internet Address) and instructions were made simple for the average person with the average computer skills. No special computer skills are required to install and use this software. The work has already been done for you in Chapter 5 which automates the process.

If you're like most of us diabetics, you have difficulty in tracking progress related to your treatment. This software not only creates a record of your blood glucose readings, but also does the math and gives your progress, daily, weekly, monthly and overall average with regard to your blood glucose levels.

It's amazing that we never realize what we are eating and when until we see it recorded. By comparing the Nutritional Information log to your blood glucose readings, your Doctor, Nutritionist, and your PharmD may get a better idea of the source of problems, if any, related to your diabetic treatment. The Nutritional Information Software creates a log to record your insulin dosages, your food intake and the exact time for each entry.

I have been a diabetic for decades. It need not be a death sentence, but it is a life threatening condition if not treated properly. Work with your life-giving team of professionals who can guide you through the sometimes difficult task of maintaining your health.

In any war, information (G-2) is the key to winning the battle. This software provides intelligence for your plan of attack. Be warned that this software, in-and-of itself will not guarantee any level of success, but may be used in conjunction with professional help to make your progress easier to track.

The scope of this book is limited to the installation and use of the special software provided. The software is only intended to enable you to more closely track your progress with regard to your nutrition, treatment and blood glucose levels.

INTRODUCTION

Prior to 1950, diabetes was far more disabling than it is today. Medical science has come a long way toward prolonging life and reducing the ill effects of this chronic condition.

Medications were not available to the extent they are today. Insulin was problematic because, what insulin there was had been derived from animal insulin. It sometimes caused sunken pock-marks or other problems at the injection site.

Technology is making the task of controlling your blood glucose levels easier to accomplish, such as the software included in this book.

The syringes were reusable glass and the needles were used for repeated injections. The diameters of the needles were larger and were less comfortable due to their size and due to their repeated use, became dull. The syringes and the needles had to be boiled in water in order to sterilize them, sometimes making the sterility of the injection less effective.

Today we have very fine needle diameters resulting in painless injections and the syringes are only used one time. They are sterile in their packages which are individually sealed at the factory. Use it once and throw it away; no more boiling and no dull needles with far less risk of infection.

Insulin is no longer derived from animals, but is Recombinant DNA, being artificially manufactured in laboratories, making them less expensive and less prone to allergic reactions at the injection site or rejection by the body's immune system.

DISCLAIMER

In today's litigious society we are all forced to take greater precautions against any misinterpretation of the obvious.

I am not a physician, and so I repeatedly recommend working with your healthcare providers in using the information gleaned from this software.

Any information regarding treatment, drugs, or other facts must be verified by your healthcare providers and is not intended to provide any course of treatment or medical advice.

I am a software engineer who has used the enclosed software for years with great success. The numbers and logs created by this software have been verified as accurate by my licensed healthcare providers who, after processing the information gleaned from the software, have concluded that the results are both accurate and helpful.

CHAPTER 1 YOUR DIET

Part of the heartache of having diabetes is the way it sometimes seems to suck up every part of your free time.

Imagine having to stop what you're doing every 4 or 5 hours and perform a ritual that involves stabbing yourself with a pin-like tool, bleeding a drop of blood, then writing down the number.

Imagine having to stop after every meal or snack to write down what you ate, how much, along with the date and time of the day.

I'm not suggesting that the diabetic not do these things, but I have automated the process so the computer is doing most of the work.

Click on the icon, write what you ate and, if you need to, enter the medication type and dosage. The computer does all the rest, entering the date and time and logging the information for you.

You can print out multiple copies if needed. I always print out 2 copies so I have one to look at while the Doctor, PharmD or Dietician is looking at theirs.

With all the times, totals, descriptions, dosages and averages laid out neatly, you have more time to talk with your healthcare professionals because they don't have to decipher your handwriting and crank through the numbers while you sit and wait.

Your progress is available at a glance.

With the cost of healthcare today, you want the maximum amount of time to work with your healthcare professional.

CHAPTER 2 KNOW YOUR ENEMY

After so many decades of being a type II diabetic, there is so much I could tell you.

There is so much I could tell you about the balance between Blood Glucose and Insulin.

There is so much I could tell you about the balance of exercise and Blood Glucose.

There is so much I could tell you about the balance of exercise and Insulin.

There is so much I could tell you about the balance of exercise and weight.

There is so much I could tell you about the balance of weight and Blood Glucose.

There is so much I could tell you about the balance of insulin and weight.

Did I mention there is a balance between weight, blood glucose, diet and exercise? It's a complex business, but I'm not a licensed Physician, so I can't tell you what I know.

I encourage you to find the answers. Your life depends on it and that's not medical advice, it's a fact.

If you have questions there are three people on your team. I will introduce each of them in the next three brief chapters.

CHAPTER 3 YOUR DIETICIAN

There are relationships between different foods that you need to be aware of.

Various foods fall into various categories, such as protein, vitamins, minerals, carbs and more.

Some of the factors in your diet include foods that metabolize at different rates. There are foods with various glycemic index levels that can cause your blood sugar readings to vary in ways you need to understand. Is a baked potato going to raise your blood sugar faster than french-fries? You might be surprised. Glycemic index and caloric values are different in the way they affect your blood sugar and weight.

Your Dietician can help you to control your blood sugar and your weight, but only if you do the work.

The entire process is much like the time I joined a gym to reduce my weight and get into shape. I paid every month faithfully weighed myself every day and never lost any weight at all. Then I figured out the problem. I had to go there and work out or the membership was useless.

My experience with Dieticians is much the same. I have studied diet and nutrition. I have visited Dieticians and had the discussions about my eating habits, but never seemed to have a lot of luck.

Then, much like the gym situation it occurred to me that knowledge of good nutrition isn't helping the situation when I'm living on spaghetti and hot dogs.

Ask your Dietician about your caloric set point and how to lower it. That will do a lot to help you control your weight.

CHAPTER 4 YOUR DOCTOR

The Doctor is your General in the war against diabetes. If you have a choice, pick a good one. Your life and health is in his hands to some extent, but only if you follow his advice.

The one person who wholly owns your success or your failure is you. No one else is usually there when you make a bad choice.

When you have the spreadsheets completed with the matrix of data depicting the averages, see how the Doctor feels about the complete overview of your measurements and information.

The matrix of average results plays in concert with the listing of meals and medications. Together they form a complete picture of your treatment, except for exercise.

You can enter your exercise information in the space provided for food, giving the distance walked or the equipment used.

Because the "Nutritional Information" log has no calculations involved, you can enter anything you want.

The log will post the time and date of the entry, but will not post the actual meal or activity time and date, so post entries as soon as possible after performing the task.

CHAPTER 5 THE PHARMD

If you're lucky enough to have a Doctor of Pharmacology assigned to you, take full advantage of their expertise. A good PharmD can advise you of the best course of treatment for you.

The PharmD is the most knowledgeable person for deciding which insulin will be best and which medications will be most effective.

When taking a blend of medications, there is a danger of interaction when some are combined in your treatment.

The PharmD is the expert on these complex interactions. Having the PharmD review your medications is a smart move.

CHAPTER 6 DOWNLOAD & INSTALL

Let's get the show on the road here. You will need your PC and an Internet connection in order to install the software covered in this course of instruction.

First you will need to prepare a place for the software and spreadsheets to go. The best place for now is probably drive C, so click on the Icon, System Information, and the list of disk drives will be displayed.

Now click on Drive C: and when it opens, right click on it. A command box will open and you will click on menu item, "New" and when the sub-folder opens, click on "Folder".

You can name the folder anything you want. I like to call it "Diabetic Software".

Bring up your Internet Browser and type in the following URL.

Be sure and type it in exactly as shown.

http://www.RobStetson.com/Diabetic/Load.html

This address is case sensitive and if you fail to capitalize the letters shown and have the rest in lower case, the connection will fail.

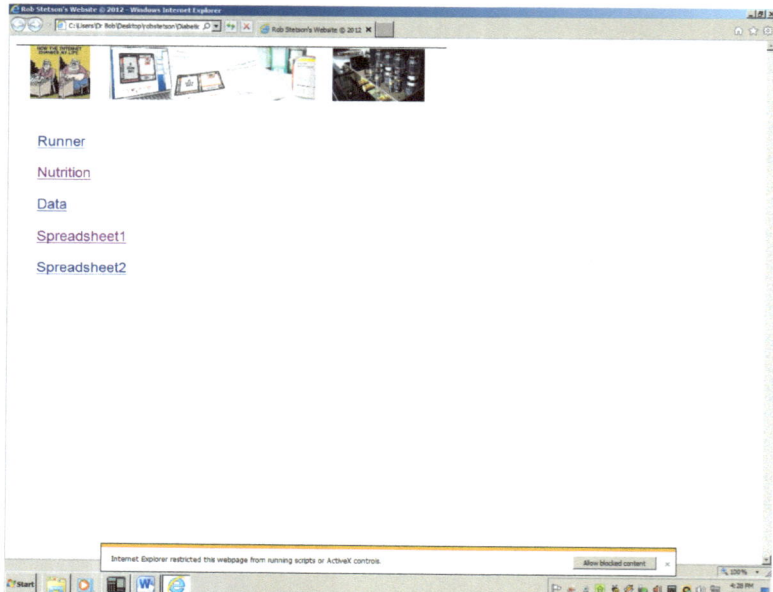

After going to the web location shown above, the screen will show a page with no menu and 5 files.

As you click on the "Runner" link, your Windows Browser will ask what you want to do with the file. Click on "Run" and be aware that this program needs to be run only once to install the DLL's for the program "Nutrition.exe". The DLL's are the "Runtime" files. There is no reason to download the program called by "Runner" unless you choose to.

I have seen warning flags for Runner saying "Unknown Publisher". Don't panic, just say,

"Yes". Saying yes just means you are allowing the program to install the runtime files needed to run the program.

After you have run the program called by the "Runner", you can install NI.exe. Click on the Link called "Nutrition" and select "Download" as your option using "Save as" and specifying C:\Diabetic\ as the target folder.

After the system has saved the file, do the same for the link, "Data", Spreadsheet1 and Spreadsheet2. With all 4 files in the folder, you have successfully installed the software.

Now you need to put an Icon on the desktop for the file NI.exe if you want to run the program conveniently.

By the way… You will find a file called z.txt in the folder. Don't delete that. It's your database which I have created in ASCII so you can read it clearly using Notepad, MS Word or any other editor.

This makes it an open source data file. I just hate it when someone writes software and then encrypts the data file so you can't get at it any other way.

I just put a shortcut to the folder on Drive C:\Diabetic\ and it enables me to not only run

NI.exe, but it also enables me to simply click on BSB1.xlsx and BSB2.xlsx.

When you click on either BSB1.xlsx or BSB2.xlsx, they open in Excel so you can read the content, print them out or enter the data.

We're going to get back to the BSB files shortly, but first, let's talk about the NI.exe file.

CHAPTER 7 USING NI.exe

When you open NI.exe the program runs with the following window as your control panel.

This control panel enables you to enter your day to day meals, readings, exercise info and medications.

Instructions are built right into the form. If you practice using the program you will become proficient at entering the data.

Notice the time and date information at the top of the form. This data is retrieved directly from your system's clock information. However accurate your system's time and date information is, that will be reflected in your data sheets.

Under the time and date box, there is a large window where you will enter the information regarding your food or exercise routine. Try to be brief. There is a lot of room to write, but the program can only scan in a certain amount of data before the buffers and arrays overflow,

Do food as one entry. Then do exercise (if you are including it) as a separate entry. When doing exercise you will have to select a mealtime for the entry because there is no exercise bullet on the list.

After you write out a meal or regimen, select one of the bullets on the left to identify the mealtime for the entry.

The bottom 2 bullets in the list of mealtime selections are for the bottom portion of the form where you enter information regarding your medication and blood sugar readings.

Since you may not be taking these readings and medications at the same time each day you are eating your meal, I have put a window toward the left under the meal cata entry window labeled "TIME". This is the time you enter with the keyboard manually.

Use the format you choose because the system does not read it, it just prints it as part of your data entries.

To the right of the "TIME" entry window is the "VALUE mg/dl" which means "Value in milligrams-per-deciliter".

That is the standard unit of blood sugar measurement.

Take the "VALUE mg/dl" straight from the window on your glucometer.

Once you have entered the time and the reading, click on the button on the far left row of buttons called "VALUE mg".

This will store the value you have entered in the window.

If you fail to put the dose in the window, and then click on the button, the values will not be stored.

Next are the 2 windows under the "VALUE mg/dl" window. These are labeled "MEDICATION DOSE 1" and "MEDICATION DOSE 2".

Once again, you have literary license to write whatever fits in the window.

If you take insulin, input the type and number of units.

If you take pills, input the type and number of pills you took.

I have 2 windows for entering data, but you can choose to leave the second one open, or you can do more medications using separate entries.

Remember, if you add more entries, clear the windows marked MEDICATION DOSE if the window is not going to be used again.

You can leave the box marked "TIME" alone if the time is still good for the additional entries.

CHAPTER 8 READING THE Z.txt FILE

NI.exe opens and uses the file Z.txt. The Z.txt file will not be created if it is not present. You will get an error when you try to run NI.exe in the absence of Z.txt.

I am going to go through the Z.txt file and explain some of the information and markers placed there by the program.

Let's look at a real file that was generated for demo purposes. This is the actual contents of a Z.txt file.

MEALS LOG

```
8/19/2011 - BREAKFAST - 3:50:38 AM    Eggs, Toas:, Coffee
8/19/2011 -      *       - 3:20 AM        Blood Sugar = 195  mg/dl
8/19/2011 -    >---      - 3:20 AM        Humalog = 12  Units
8/19/2011 -    >---      - 3:20 AM     Humalin N = 82  Units
8/19/2011 -      *       - 9:38 AM        Blood Sugar = 201  mg/dl
8/19/2011 -    >---      - 938 AM       Humalog = 6  Units
8/19/2011 -      *       - 5:08 PM        Blood Sugar = 158  mg/dl
8/19/2011 -    >---      - 5:08 PM     Humalog = 12  Units
8/19/2011 -    >---      - 5:08 PM     Humalin N = 84  Units
8/19/2011  - DINNER      - 11:02:25 PM     STEAK, POTATO,
STRING BEANS
8/20/2011 - SNACK        - 2:30:27 AM    Coffee
8/20/2011 -      *       - 4:42 AM        Blood Sugar = 140  mg/dl
8/20/2011 -    >---      - 4:42 AM     Humalin N = 82  Units
8/20/2011 - BREAKFAST - 6:54:45 AM    Eggs, Bread, Grits, Coffee
8/20/2011 -    >---      - 6:55 AM       Humalog = 15  Units
8/20/2011 -      *       - 12:36 PM       Blood Sugar = 155  mg/dl
8/20/2011 -      *       - 5:30 PM        Blood Sugar = 160  mg/dl
8/20/2011 - DINNER      - 5:55:43 PM     STEAK, POTATO, STRING
BEANS
8/20/2011 -    >---      - 6:01 PM       Humalog = 15  Units
8/20/2011 -    >---      - 6:01 PM     Humalin N = 182  Units
8/20/2011  - SNACK      - 7:40:09 PM      DONUT, SOUTHERN
COMFORT, DIET SPRITE
8/20/2011 - SNACK       - 11:32:30 PM    PIZZA
8/21/2011 -    >---      - 1:40 AM       Humalog = 5  Units
8/21/2011 -      *       - 6:42 AM        Blood Sugar = 151  mg/dl
8/21/2011 -    >---      - 6:42 AM     Humalin N = 82  Units
8/21/2011 - SNACK       - 6:48:44 AM    COFFEE
8/21/2011 - BREAKFAST - 8:45:21 AM    eggs, bacon, bread, coffee
8/21/2011 -    >---      - 8:46 AM       Humalog = 15  Units
```

8/21/2011 -   *   - 12:14 PM   Blood Sugar = 87 mg/dl
8/21/2011 - DINNER   - 3:06:51 PM   Steak, Potato, Salad, Bread
8/21/2011 -   *   - 8:52 PM   Blood Sugar = 334 mg/dl
8/21/2011 -   >---   - 9:18 PM   Humalog = 15 Units
8/21/2011 -   >---   - 9:18 PM   Humalin N = 82 Units
8/21/2011 - SNACK   - 9:34 PM   JACK DANIELS, DIET SPRITE
8/22/2011 - SNACK   - 3:16:29 AM   PIECE OF CHOCOLATE
8/22/2011 - BREAKFAST - 8:17:14 AM   COFFEE, 2-DOENUTS
8/22/2011 -   *   - 12:30 PM   Blood Sugar = 239 mg/dl

Now let's look at the file after being printed;

MEALS LOG

8/19/201 1 - BREAKFAST - 3:50:38 AM   Eggs, Toast, Coffee
            *   - 3:20   AM   Blood Sugar = 195 mg/dl
           >---   - 3:20   AM   Humalog = 12 Units
           >---   - 3:20   AM   Humalin N = 82 Units
            *   - 9:38   AM   Blood Sugar = 201 mg/dl
           >---   - 938   AM   Humalog = 6 Units
            *   - 5:08 PM   Blood Sugar = 158 mg/dl
           >---   - 5:08 PM   Humalog = 12 Units
           >---   - 5:08 PM   Humalin N = 84 Units
        DINNER   - 1 1:02:25 PM   STEAK, POTATO, STRING BEANS

8/20/201 1 - SNACK   - 2:30:27 AM   Coffee
            *   - 4:42   AM   Blood Sugar = 140 mg/dl
           >---   - 4:42   AM   Humalin N = 82 Units
        BREAKFAST - 6:54:45 AM   Eggs, Bread, Grits, Coffee
           >---   - 6:55   AM   Humalog = 15 Units
            *   - 12:36 PM   Blood Sugar = 155 mg/dl
            *   - 5:30 PM   Blood Sugar = 160 mg/dl
        DINNER   - 5:55:43 PM   STEAK, POT ATO, STRING BEANS
           >---   - 6:01 PM   Humalog = 15 Units
           >---   - 6:01 PM   Humalin N = 182 Units
        SNACK   - 7:40:09 PM   DOENUT , SOUTHERN COMFORT, DIET SPRITE
        SNACK   - 1 1:32:30 PM   PIZZA

8/21/201 1 -   >---   - 1:40 AM   Humalog = 5 Units
            *   - 6:42   AM   Blood Sugar = 151 mg/dl
           >---   - 6:42   AM   Humalin N = 82 Units
        SNACK   - 6:48:44 AM   COFFEE
        BREAKFAST - 8:45:21 AM   eggs, bacon, bread, coffee
           >---   - 8:46   AM   Humalog = 15 Units
            *   - 12:14 PM   Blood Sugar = 87 mg/dl
        DINNER   - 3:06:51 PM   Steak, Potato, Salad, Bread
            *   - 8:52 PM   Blood Sugar = 334 mg/dl
           >---   - 9:18 PM   Humalog = 15 Units
           >---   - 9:18 PM   Humalin N = 82 Units
        SNACK   - 9:34 PM   JACK DANIELS, DIET SPRITE

8/22/201 1 - SNACK   - 3:16:29 AM   PIECE OF CHOCHOLATE
        BREAKFAST - 8:17:14 AM   COFFEE, 2-DOENUTS
            *   - 12:30 PM   Blood Sugar = 239 mg/dl

You will notice that there is an empty line and a horizontal line beginning each new day in the printout above. The software

inserts these during the printing process. These empty lines and the horizontal line separating the days are not present in the data file itself.

They are there to make the report easier to read. Also, during the printing process, the software injects pagination to ensure that if the pages ever get separated, they can be reassembled in their correct order.

Each entry is identified in the actual file by either the name of the meal or the other types of entries.

Medication is flagged by the ">---" symbols.

Blood sugar readings are flagged by the asterisk, "*".

This makes it easier to pick out the data points that you might be looking for in the data.

CHAPTER 9 USING THE BSBs

You see the ads on TV and they all say, "Test your readings and test them often."

"Often" is rather subjective, so let me say, "Test your readings and test them in the specific frequencies required by your health care provider."

The pre-formulated Excel Spread Sheet will give you a running total of your readings along with a running average for breakfast, lunch, and dinner. It will also give an average trend for mornings, noon and evening readings. It also gives an average trend daily, weekly and total over all.

By seeing your average trends, you can consult your Nutritional Information log printed out from (Z.txt) and, hopefully, get some clues to the changes in your average readings.

The Excel formulas are not complex and they do the entire calculation for you. The formulas are already embedded in the spreadsheets when you download them.

There is a row and a column that requires no formulation. These have an open labeling format requirement, meaning that you can type in anything you want.

I have typed in the first row that will appear at the top of the page when you decide to print them out.

The left column "A" is the day of the week and I insert the month number 1 through 12, a slash and the days date for each row. You can see the method I use in the example screenshots.

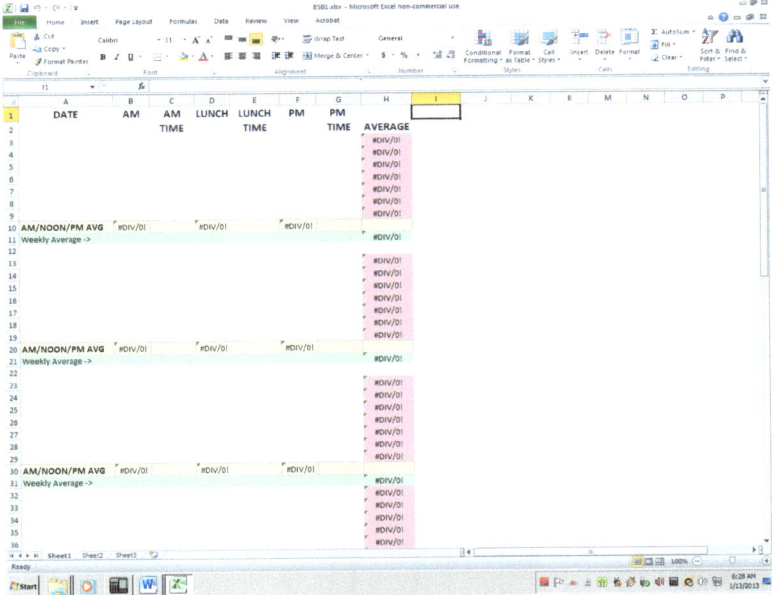

Above is the 3 readings a day spreadsheet.

Below is the 4 readings a day spreadsheet.

Both are essentially the same in terms of the formulation and the daily averages.

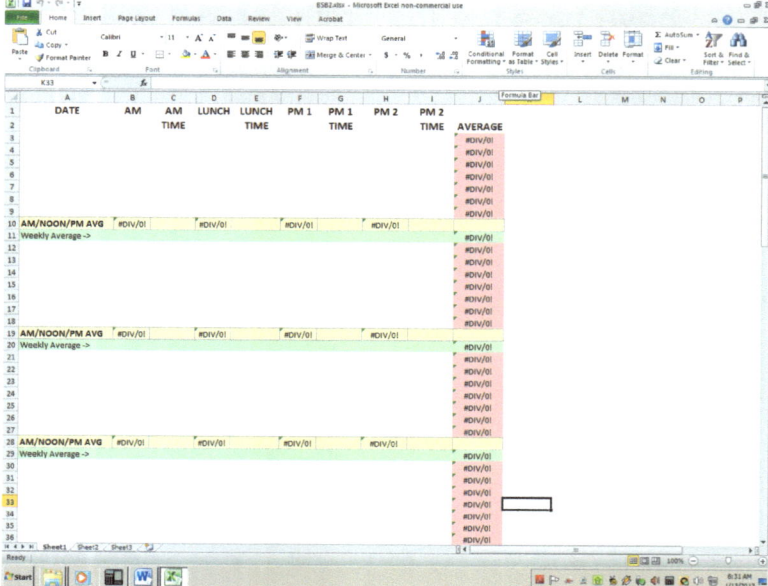

The spreadsheet shown above is the way it will look when you download the software for the first time.

The empty spreadsheet is clustered with the content "#REF!" which means there is no data available for the formula.

You will be providing data as you take your readings.

Some of the examples shown here have three columns for data and some have four columns for data. I have provided both sizes of forms because some people measure three times a day and others measure four times a day.

DATE		AM	AM TIME	LUNCH	LUNCH TIME	PM 1	PM 1 TIME	FM 2	PM 2 TIME	AVERAGE
SUN	11/18	117	4:57 AM	122	11:32 AM	121	5:48 PM			120.00
MON	11/19	162	4:25 AM	173	12:05 PM	114	5:53 PM	119	8:59 PM	142.00
TUES	11/20	127	4:59 AM	145	11:37 AM			123	11:19 PM	131.67
WED	11/21	108	4:57 AM	123	11:36 AM	152	5:25 PM			127.67
THURS	11/22	146	8:38 AM	138	1:48 PM	120	5:23 PM			134.67
FRI	11/23	148	5:30 AM	75	11:42 AM			101	8:08 PM	108.00
SAT	11/24	136	5:06 AM	119	12:04 PM			100	8:21 PM	118.33
AM/NOON/PM AVG		135		128		127		111		
Weekly Average ->										125
SUN	11/25	112	6:08 AM	85	11:31 AM	132	5:04 PM	112	7:25 PM	110.25
MON	11/26	120	5:12 AM	120	1:26 PM	132	6:33 PM	123	8:36 PM	110.25
TUES	11/27	118	5:07 AM	149	2:26 PM	153	5:09 PM	110	7:11 PM	132.50
WED	11/28	100	4:32 AM	101	11:28 AM	115	5:18 PM	117	9:05 PM	108.25
THURS	11/29	136	7:59 AM	139	12:29 PM	73	4:51 PM	127	7:53 PM	118.75
FRI	11/30	137	5:24 AM	95	1:56 PM	131	5:00 PM	137	7:53 PM	125.00
SAT	12/1	112	4:55 AM	132	2:05 PM	109	6:14 PM			117.67
AM/NOON/PM AVG		119		117		121		121		
Weekly Average ->										120
SUN	12/2	117	5:30 AM	112	12:22 PM	155	6:13 PM	134	8:34 PM	129.50
MON	12/3	138	5:31 AM	112	12:07 PM	179	4:50 PM	122	6:09 PM	137.75
TUES	12/4	102	7:46 AM	127	3:20 PM	172	7:51 PM	113	9:21 PM	128.50
WED	12/5	119	9:03 AM	72	2:39 PM			131	7:26 PM	107.33
THURS	12/6	132	8:25 AM	136	12:11 PM	157	6:20 PM	119	9:54 PM	136.00
FRI	12/7	135	9:04 AM	119	12:02 PM	157	6:20 PM	129	8:54 PM	135.00
SAT	12/8	110	6:50 AM	95	1:22 PM			110	10:10 PM	105.00
SUN	12/9	122	6:26 AM	91	1:16 PM	189	5:41 PM	117	8:00 PM	129.75
MON	12/10	131	4:57 AM	95	11:01 AM					113.00
AM/NOON/PM AVG		123		107		168		122		
Weekly Average ->										130
ALL READINGS		126		117		139		118		125

The spreadsheet shown above is an example of a sheet that has been filled out with readings and has all the averages in place. The averages appear automatically as you enter each new entry.

When you are done with the spreadsheet, you can erase the contents by placing the mouse pointer on the upper left hand corner of each set of data fields and dragging it down and to the right until all the data fields are grey and then right clicking on the mouse.

The menu appears and you select, "Clear Contents" to erase the old data and it's ready for you to fill out the new form.

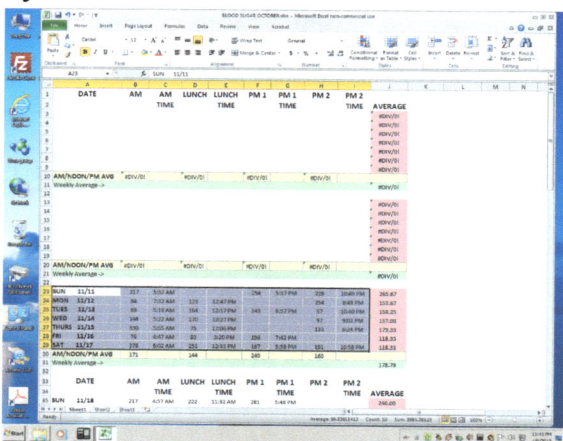

Be very careful not to erase the areas of the spreadsheet that contain all of the automatic averaging values, as these areas contain the formulas needed for the form to work.

Across the bottom of each week there is a yellow bar showing the morning, noontime and evening readings for each week.

Each week is terminated by a green bar across the bottom of the week. The green bar is located just below the yellow bar showing the morning, noontime and evening readings. The weekly average appears just before the daily averages.

Down the right we have a pink band with the daily averages for each day of the week.

All average calculations are the "Mean Averages".

The two spreadsheets shown below have the orange bar at the bottom of the sheet so you can see the area where the total overall average is displayed.

These total overall averages are given for the morning, noontime and either 1 or 2 evening readings depending on which spreadsheet you are using.

The average reading given at the far right end of the orange band is the total overall average reading for the entire array of values you have put into the spreadsheet.

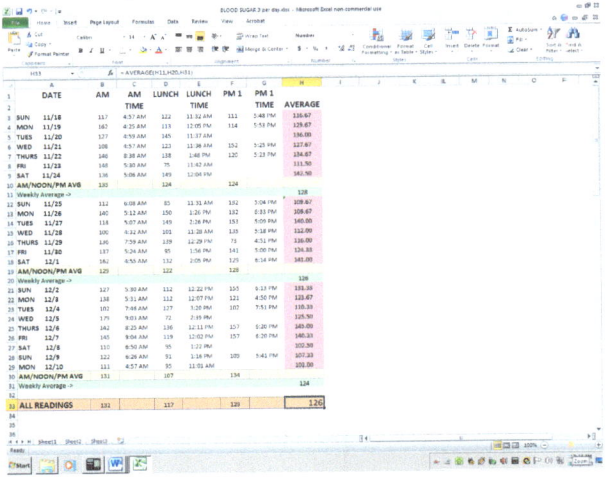

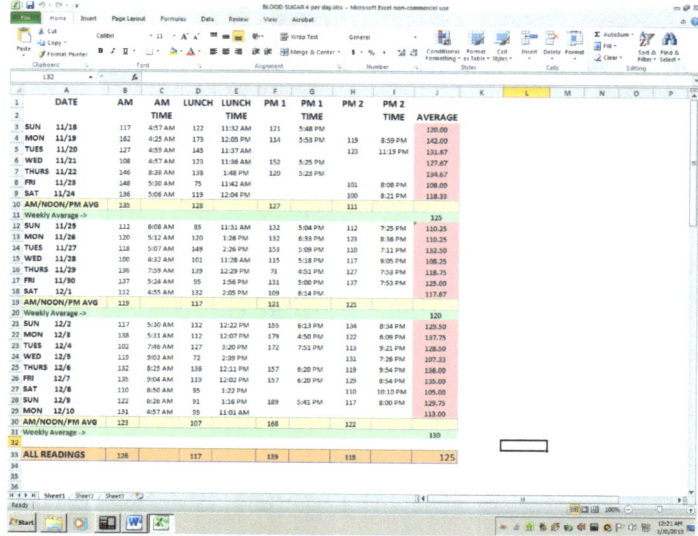

On the 2 Excel Spreadsheets above we have an example of a cluster of readings taken over a three week period.

EXCEL FORMULAS

For those of you who are interested in the various formulas we have entered into both of the spreadsheets, I am including this information here. It will also be of value if you want to make your own variation of the two given in this book.

To start with, the areas where you enter your readings and the time have no formulas associated with them. They are just raw values entered from the keyboard.

1. Down the right hand side of each matrix

=AVERAGE(B6,D6,F6,H6)

Where "=" declares a formula is to be entered. "AVERAGE" defines the function "SUM" of all data divided by "NUMBER" of all data, where Xn,Xn,Xn,Xn are the Cartesian coordinates of the data elements.

2. Down the column for each item in the data block.

=AVERAGE(B3:B9)

Where "=" declares a formula is to be entered. "AVERAGE" defines the function "SUM" of all data divided by "NUMBER" of all data, where Xn:Xn are the span of Cartesian coordinates of the data elements.

3. In the lower right hand corner of each matrix

=AVERAGE(B10,D10,F10,H10)

Where "=" declares a formula is to be entered. "AVERAGE" defines the function "SUM" of all data divided by "NUMBER" of all data, where Xn,Xn,Xn,Xn are the Cartesian coordinates of the data elements.

4. Across the orange band at the end of the matrixes

=AVERAGE(B10,B19,B30)

Where "=" declares a formula is to be entered. "AVERAGE" defines the function "SUM" of all data divided by "NUMBER" of all data, where Xn,Xn,Xn,Xn are the Cartesian coordinates of the data elements.

5. In the far right hand lowest corner of the last page, the grand total average matrix

= AVERAGE(J11,J20,J31,J40)

Where "=" declares a formula is to be entered. "AVERAGE" defines the function "SUM" of all data divided by "NUMBER" of all data, where Xn,Xn,Xn,Xn are the Cartesian coordinates of the sum average totals for each data block.

CHAPTER 10 SOURCE CODE

The following is the source code for the Nutritional Information tracker;

First we have the "Form";

And we have the "Form Source Code;

```
VERSION 5.00
Begin VB.Form Form1
    Caption     = "Nutritional Information        By
Robert Stetson"
    ClientHeight  = 6870
    ClientLeft  = 120
    ClientTop   = 420
```

```
ClientWidth    =  6375
LinkTopic      =  "Form1"
ScaleHeight    =  6870
ScaleWidth     =  6375
StartUpPosition =  3  'Windows Default
Begin VB.TextBox Text7
   Height      =  375
   Left        =  4560
   TabIndex    =  20
   Top         =  5280
   Width       =  1575
End
Begin VB.OptionButton Option6
   Caption     =  "Insulin"
   Height      =  495
   Left        =  120
   TabIndex    =  18
   Top         =  3720
   Width       =  1095
End
Begin VB.TextBox Text6
   Height      =  405
   Left        =  4560
   TabIndex    =  17
   Top         =  4800
   Width       =  1575
End
Begin VB.TextBox Text4
   Height      =  375
   Left        =  4560
   TabIndex    =  13
   Top         =  4320
   Width       =  1695
End
Begin VB.TextBox Text3
   Height      =  375
   Left        =  1320
```

```
    TabIndex    =  12
    Top         =  4320
    Width       =  1335
End
Begin VB.OptionButton Option5
    Caption     =  "Blood Sgr"
    Height      =  375
    Left        =  120
    TabIndex    =  11
    Top         =  3240
    Width       =  1095
End
Begin VB.TextBox Text2
    Alignment   =  2  'Center
    Height      =  405
    Left        =  1200
    TabIndex    =  9
    Top         =  840
    Width       =  5055
End
Begin VB.CommandButton Command4
    Caption     =  "EXIT"
    Height      =  495
    Left        =  3360
    TabIndex    =  8
    Top         =  6240
    Width       =  3015
End
Begin VB.CommandButton Command3
    Caption     =  "PRINT"
    Height      =  495
    Left        =  360
    TabIndex    =  7
    Top         =  6240
    Width       =  2895
End
Begin VB.OptionButton Option4
```

```
      Caption      =  "Snack"
      Height      =  255
      Left       =  120
      TabIndex     =  6
      Top        =  2880
      Width       =  1095
   End
   Begin VB.OptionButton Option3
      Caption      =  "Dinner"
      Height      =  375
      Left       =  120
      TabIndex     =  5
      Top        =  2400
      Width       =  1095
   End
   Begin VB.OptionButton Option2
      Caption      =  "Lunch"
      Height      =  375
      Left       =  120
      TabIndex     =  4
      Top        =  1920
      Width       =  1095
   End
   Begin VB.OptionButton Option1
      Caption      =  "Breakfast"
      Height      =  375
      Left       =  120
      TabIndex     =  3
      Top        =  1440
      Width       =  1095
   End
   Begin VB.TextBox Text1
      Height      =  2895
      Left       =  1200
      TabIndex     =  2
      Top        =  1320
      Width       =  5055
```

```
End
Begin VB.Label Label8
   Alignment     =  1  'Right Justify
   Caption       =  "HUMALIN N INSULIN"
   Height        =  255
   Left          =  2760
   TabIndex      =  19
   Top           =  5400
   Width         =  1695
End
Begin VB.Label Label7
   Alignment     =  1  'Right Justify
   Caption       =  "HUMALOG INSULIN"
   Height        =  255
   Left          =  2760
   TabIndex      =  16
   Top           =  4920
   Width         =  1695
End
Begin VB.Label Label5
   Alignment     =  1  'Right Justify
   Caption       =  "VALUE mg/dl"
   Height        =  255
   Left          =  3240
   TabIndex      =  15
   Top           =  4440
   Width         =  1215
End
Begin VB.Label Label4
   Alignment     =  1  'Right Justify
   Caption       =  "TIME"
   Height        =  255
   Left          =  240
   TabIndex      =  14
   Top           =  4440
   Width         =  975
End
```

```
Begin VB.Label Label3
   Caption     = "  ENTER MEAL INFORMATION FIRST
- - - THEN SELECT MEAL TYPE ON LEFT"
   Height      = 255
   Left        = 120
   TabIndex    = 10
   Top         = 5880
   Width       = 6135
End
Begin VB.Label Label2
   Caption     = "Time & Date"
   Height      = 255
   Index       = 0
   Left        = 120
   TabIndex    = 1
   Top         = 960
   Width       = 1935
End
Begin VB.Label Label1
   Alignment   = 2 'Center
   Caption     = "Nutritional Informatior"
   BeginProperty Font
     Name          = "Arial"
     Size          = 24
     Charset       = 0
     Weight        = 700
     Underline     = 0 'False
     Italic        = 0 'False
     Strikethrough = 0 'False
   EndProperty
   Height      = 615
   Left        = 120
   TabIndex    = 0
   Top         = 120
   Width       = 6135
 End
End
```

```
Attribute VB_Name = "Form1"
Attribute VB_GlobalNameSpace = False
Attribute VB_Creatable = False
Attribute VB_PredeclaredId = True
Attribute VB_Exposed = False
Dim A$                          ' System Time
Dim b$                          ' System Date
Dim c$                          ' Entry Identifier
Dim d As String                  ' Date read in from the
disk
Dim S$                          ' Print a line without the
redundant date
Dim lines As Integer             ' Counter for the
printed page lines
Dim pages As Integer             ' Counter for the
printed page numbers
Dim same As String               ' Flag used to
suppress the redundant date field
Dim L As Integer                 ' For Next and Loop
Counter to track array locations
Dim counter As Integer           ' Counter for
reading data from the disk
Dim source As String             ' Data Input line
length
Dim hold() As String             ' Array identifier
Option Explicit                  'Require all Variable
Declarations
Private Sub Command3_Click()
' *********************************** PRINT
***********************************
Open "z.txt" For Input As #1          ' Open data file
for input
Printer.Font.Name = "Times New Roman"      ' Set
Font Size and Style
Printer.Font.Size = 10
lines = 1                         ' Initialize Pagination
pages = 1
```

```
                                    ' Print Page Number
        Printer.Print "                    " & "PAGE " & pages
        Do Until (EOF(1))                ' Grow the array
until complete
                                    ' Format Top of the Page
        If lines = 1 Then Printer.Print
        If lines = 1 Then Printer.Print
        If lines = 1 Then Printer.Print
        If lines = 1 Then Printer.Print
        If lines = 1 Then Printer.Print
        If lines = 1 Then Printer.Print
        If lines = 1 Then Printer.Print
        If lines = 1 Then Printer.Print
        If lines = 1 Then lines = lines + 9        ' Resynchronize
Pagination
        lines = lines + 1
        If lines = 50 Then pages = pages + 1        ' Increment
Page Numbers
        Line Input #1, source                ' Read in next
entry
                                    ' Print Date only once a day
        d = Left(source, 4)
        L = Len(source)
        If Left(source, 4) = same And source <> "" Then S$ = "
" & Mid(source, 12, (L - 11))
        If same <> d And Left(source, 4) <> "    " Then
Printer.Print "                " &
"
_____
_____"
        If same <> d Then Printer.Print "                    " &
source
        If same = d Then Printer.Print "                    "; S$
                                    ' Start new page after 50
lines
        If lines = 50 Then Printer.NewPage
        If lines = 50 Then Printer.Print "                    " &
"PAGE " & pages
```

```
        If lines = 50 Then lines = 1              ' Restart line
counter on new page
        same = d                    ' Reset new date
detector
        Loop
        Printer.EndDoc                  ' Force printer to
start print immediately
        Close #1                    ' Close the data file
        End Sub

        Private Sub Command4_Click()
        Close                   ' Close all open files
        End                 ' Close out the
application
        End Sub

        Private Sub Form_Load()                 ' Load the
Application Window to the desktop
        A$ = Time
        b$ = Date
        Text2 = "************ ENTER MEAL INFO" & " - " & A$
& " - " & b$ & " *****************"
        counter = 0
        Open "z.txt" For Input As #1                ' Open the data
file
        Do Until (EOF(1))               ' Read the data file
until the end
        counter = counter + 1               ' Add a line
        Line Input #1, source               ' Read in next
entry=
        ReDim Preserve hold(counter)                ' Grow the
array until complete
        hold(counter) = source              ' Write new data
to the array
        Loop
        Close #1                    ' Close data file when
the array is loaded
```

```
End Sub

Private Sub Option1_Click()
c$ = "BREAKFAST"
A$ = Time
b$ = Date
Open "z.txt" For Output As #1
counter = counter + 1                          ' Add a line
Text2 = b$ & " - " & c$ & " - " & A$
ReDim Preserve hold(counter)                   ' grow the
data array
hold(counter) = b$ & " - " & c$ & " - " & A$ & "    " &
Text1
For L = 1 To counter
Print #1, hold(L)                    ' Write the new data
line to the disk
Next L

Close #1

End Sub

Private Sub Option2_Click()
c$ = "LUNCH       "
A$ = Time
b$ = Date
Open "z.txt" For Output As #1
counter = counter + 1                          ' Add a line
Text2 = b$ & " - " & c$ & " - " & A$
ReDim Preserve hold(counter)                   ' grow the
data array
hold(counter) = b$ & " - " & c$ & " - " & A$ & "    " &
Text1
For L = 1 To counter
Print #1, hold(L)                    ' Write the new data
line to the disk
Next L
```

```
        Close #1
        End Sub

        Private Sub Option3_Click()
        c$ = "DINNER      "
        A$ = Time
        b$ = Date
        Open "z.txt" For Output As #1
        counter = counter + 1                    ' Add a line
        Text2 = b$ & " - " & c$ & " - " & A$
        ReDim Preserve hold(counter)                  ' grow the
data array
        hold(counter) = b$ & " - " & c$ & " - " & A$ & "    " &
Text1
        For L = 1 To counter
        Print #1, hold(L)                    ' Write the new data
line to the disk
        Next L

        Close #1
        End Sub

        Private Sub Option4_Click()
        c$ = "SNACK       "
        A$ = Time
        b$ = Date
        Open "z.txt" For Output As #1
        counter = counter + 1                    ' Add a line
        Text2 = b$ & " - " & c$ & " - " & A$
        ReDim Preserve hold(counter)                  ' grow the
data array
        hold(counter) = b$ & " - " & c$ & " - " & A$ & "    " &
Text1
        For L = 1 To counter
        Print #1, hold(L)                    ' Write the new data
line to the disk
```

```
        Next L

        Close #1

        End Sub

        Private Sub Option5_Click()
        c$ = "     *              "
        A$ = Text3
        b$ = Date
        Open "z.txt" For Output As #1
        counter = counter + 1                    ' Add a line
        Text2 = b$ & " - " & c$ & " - " & A$
        ReDim Preserve hold(counter)             ' grow the
data array
        hold(counter) = b$ & " - " & c$ & " - " & A$ & "
Blood Sugar = " & Text4 & "  mg/dl"
        For L = 1 To counter
        Print #1, hold(L)                        ' Write the new data
line to the disk
        Next L

        Close #1

        End Sub

        Private Sub Option6_Click()

        c$ = "    >---            "
        A$ = Text3
        b$ = Date
        If Text6 <> "" Then Open "z.txt" For Output As #1  '
Open Data file only if data is present
        If Text6 <> "" Then counter = counter + 1       ' Add a
line
        If Text6 <> "" Then Text2 = b$ & " - " & c$ & " - " & A$
```

41

```
        If Text6 <> "" Then ReDim Preserve hold(counter)    '
grow the data array
        If Text6 <> "" Then hold(counter) = b$ & " - " & c$ & " - "
& A$ & "     Humalog = " & Text6 & "  Units"
        For L = 1 To counter
        If Text6 <> "" Then Print #1, hold(L)           ' Write the
new data line to the disk if present
        Next L
        Close #1                        ' Close Data File
        If Text7 <> "" Then Open "z.txt" For Output As #1   '
Open Data file only if data is present
        If Text7 <> "" Then counter = counter + 1        ' Add a
line
        If Text7 <> "" Then Text2 = b$ & " - " & c$ & " - " & A$
        If Text7 <> "" Then ReDim Preserve hold(counter)    '
grow the data array
        If Text7 <> "" Then hold(counter) = b$ & " - " & c$ & " - "
& A$ & "    Humalin N = " & Text7 & "  Units"
        For L = 1 To counter
        If Text7 <> "" Then Print #1, hold(L)          ' Write the
new data line to the disk if present
        Next L
        Close #1                        ' Close Data File
        End Sub
```

And we have the Executable Source Code;

```
        Dim A$                  ' System Time
        Dim b$                  ' System Date
        Dim c$                  ' Entry Identifier
        Dim d As String            ' Date read in from the
disk
        Dim S$                     ' Print a line without the
redundant date
        Dim lines As Integer            ' Counter for the
printed page lines
```

```
        Dim pages As Integer                    ' Counter for the
printed page numbers
        Dim same As String                      ' Flag used to
suppress the redundant date field
        Dim L As Integer                        ' For Next and Loop
Counter to track array locations
        Dim counter As Integer                  ' Counter for
reading data from the disk
        Dim source As String                    ' Data input line
length
        Dim hold() As String                    ' Array identifier
        Option Explicit                        'Require all Variable
Declarations
        Private Sub Command3_Click()
        ' ********************************* PRINT
**********************************
        Open "z.txt" For Input As #1            ' Open data file
for input
        Printer.Font.Name = "Times New Roman"       ' Set
Font Size and Style
        Printer.Font.Size = 10
        lines = 1                               ' Initialize Pagination
        pages = 1
                                                ' Print Page Number
        Printer.Print "                " & "PAGE " & pages
        Do Until (EOF(1))                       ' Grow the array
until complete
                                                ' Format Top of the Page
        If lines = 1 Then Printer.Print
        If lines = 1 Then Printer.Print
        If lines = 1 Then Printer.Print
        If lines = 1 Then Printer.Print
        If lines = 1 Then Printer.Print
        If lines = 1 Then Printer.Print
        If lines = 1 Then Printer.Print
        If lines = 1 Then Printer.Print
```

```
        If lines = 1 Then lines = lines + 9          ' Resynchronize
Pagination
        lines = lines + 1
        If lines = 50 Then pages = pages + 1          ' Increment
Page Numbers
        Line Input #1, source                ' Read in next
entry
                                        ' Print Date only once a day
        d = Left(source, 4)
        L = Len(source)
        If Left(source, 4) = same And source <> "" Then S$ = "
" & Mid(source, 12, (L - 11))
        If same <> d And Left(source, 4) <> "   " Then
Printer.Print "                "  &
"_____
_____"
        If same <> d Then Printer.Print "                     " &
source
        If same = d Then Printer.Print "                     "; S$
                                ' Start new page after 50
lines
        If lines = 50 Then Printer.NewPage
        If lines = 50 Then Printer.Print "                     " &
"PAGE " & pages
        If lines = 50 Then lines = 1          ' Restart line
counter on new page
        same = d                      ' Reset new date
detector
        Loop
        Printer.EndDoc                  ' Force printer to
start print immediately
        Close #1                      ' Close the data file
        End Sub

        Private Sub Command4_Click()
        Close                         ' Close all open files
```

```
        End                             ' Close out the
application
        End Sub

        Private Sub Form_Load()              ' Load the
Application Window to the desktop
        A$ = Time
        b$ = Date
        Text2 = "************ ENTER MEAL INFO ' & " - " & A$
& " - " & b$ & " *****************"
        counter = 0
        Open "z.txt" For Input As #1           ' Open the data
file
        Do Until (EOF(1))                  ' Read the data file
until the end
        counter = counter + 1              ' Add a line
        Line Input #1, source              ' Read in next
entry=
        ReDim Preserve hold(counter)            ' Grow the
array until complete
        hold(counter) = source             ' Write new data
to the array
        Loop
        Close #1                        ' Close data file when
the array is loaded
        End Sub

        Private Sub Option1_Click()
        c$ = "BREAKFAST"
        A$ = Time
        b$ = Date
        Open "z.txt" For Output As #1
        counter = counter + 1              ' Add a line
        Text2 = b$ & " - " & c$ & " - " & A$
        ReDim Preserve hold(counter)            ' grow the
data array
```

45

```
        hold(counter) = b$ & " - " & c$ & " - " & A$ & "     " &
Text1
        For L = 1 To counter
        Print #1, hold(L)                    ' Write the new data
line to the disk
        Next L

        Close #1

        End Sub

        Private Sub Option2_Click()
        c$ = "LUNCH       "
        A$ = Time
        b$ = Date
        Open "z.txt" For Output As #1
        counter = counter + 1                ' Add a line
        Text2 = b$ & " - " & c$ & " - " & A$
        ReDim Preserve hold(counter)              ' grow the
data array
        hold(counter) = b$ & " - " & c$ & " - " & A$ & "     " &
Text1
        For L = 1 To counter
        Print #1, hold(L)                    ' Write the new data
line to the disk
        Next L

        Close #1
        End Sub

        Private Sub Option3_Click()
        c$ = "DINNER      "
        A$ = Time
        b$ = Date
        Open "z.txt" For Output As #1
        counter = counter + 1                ' Add a line
        Text2 = b$ & " - " & c$ & " - " & A$
```

```
        ReDim Preserve hold(counter)              ' grow the
data array
        hold(counter) = b$ & " - " & c$ & " - " & A$ & "     " &
Text1
        For L = 1 To counter
        Print #1, hold(L)                        ' Write the new data
line to the disk
        Next L

        Close #1
        End Sub

        Private Sub Option4_Click()
        c$ = "SNACK       "
        A$ = Time
        b$ = Date
        Open "z.txt" For Output As #1
        counter = counter + 1                    ' Add a line
        Text2 = b$ & " - " & c$ & " - " & A$
        ReDim Preserve hold(counter)                ' grow the
data array
        hold(counter) = b$ & " - " & c$ & " - " & A$ & "     " &
Text1
        For L = 1 To counter
        Print #1, hold(L)                        ' Write the new data
line to the disk
        Next L

        Close #1

        End Sub

        Private Sub Option5_Click()
        c$ = "    *            "
        A$ = Text3
        b$ = Date
        Open "z.txt" For Output As #1
```

```
        counter = counter + 1                    ' Add a line
        Text2 = b$ & " - " & c$ & " - " & A$
        ReDim Preserve hold(counter)             ' grow the
data array
        hold(counter) = b$ & " - " & c$ & " - " & A$ & "
Blood Sugar = " & Text4 & "  mg/dl"
        For L = 1 To counter
        Print #1, hold(L)                    ' Write the new data
line to the disk
        Next L


        Close #1


        End Sub


        Private Sub Option6_Click()


        c$ = "    >---            "
        A$ = Text3
        b$ = Date
        If Text6 <> "" Then Open "z.txt" For Output As #1   '
Open Data file only if data is present
        If Text6 <> "" Then counter = counter + 1       ' Add a
line
        If Text6 <> "" Then Text2 = b$ & " - " & c$ & " - " & A$
        If Text6 <> "" Then ReDim Preserve hold(counter)   '
grow the data array
        If Text6 <> "" Then hold(counter) = b$ & " - " & c$ & " - "
& A$ & "     Humalog = " & Text6 & "  Units"
        For L = 1 To counter
        If Text6 <> "" Then Print #1, hold(L)            ' Write the
new data line to the disk if present
        Next L
        Close #1                        ' Close Data File
        If Text7 <> "" Then Open "z.txt" For Output As #1   '
Open Data file only if data is present
```

```
        If Text7 <> "" Then counter = counter + 1          ' Add a
line
        If Text7 <> "" Then Text2 = b$ & " - " & c$ & " - " & A$
        If Text7 <> "" Then ReDim Preserve hold(ccunter)    '
grow the data array
        If Text7 <> "" Then hold(counter) = b$ & " - " & c$ & " - "
& A$ & "    Humalin N = " & Text7 & "  Units"
        For L = 1 To counter
        If Text7 <> "" Then Print #1, hold(L)           ' Write the
new data line to the disk if present
        Next L
        Close #1                              ' Close Data File
        End Sub
```

www.ingramcontent.com/pod-product-compliance
Lightning Source LLC
Chambersburg PA
CBHW040745010626
45792CB00027B/257